The Healing Power of Fruit

Using Fruit to Cure Yourself Naturally

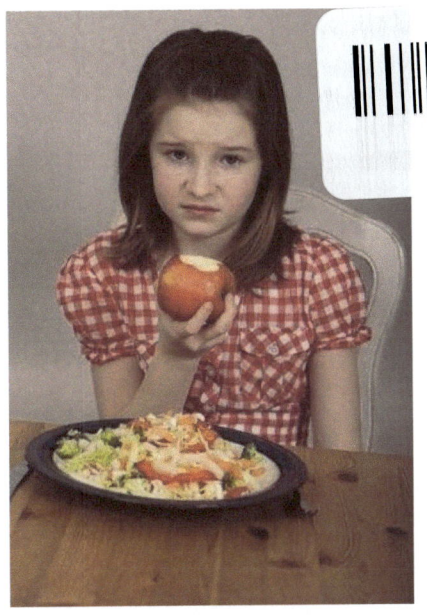

Dueep Jyot Singh

Healthy Living Series

Mendon Cottage Books

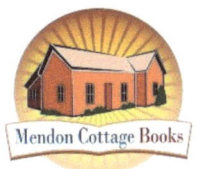

JD-Biz Publishing

Disclaimer

The information is this book is provided for informational purposes only. It is not intended to be used and medical advice or a substitute for proper medical treatment by a qualified health care provider. The information is believed to be accurate as presented based on research by the author.

The contents have not been evaluated by the U.S. Food and Drug Administration or any other Government or Health Organization and the contents in this book are not to be used to treat cure or prevent disease.

The author or publisher is not responsible for the use or safety of any diet, procedure or treatment mentioned in this book. The author or publisher is not responsible for errors or omissions that may exist.

Warning

The Book is for informational purposes only and before taking on any diet, treatment or medical procedure, it is recommended to consult with your primary health care provider.

Our books are available at

1. Amazon.com

2. Barnes and Noble

3. Itunes

4. Kobo

5. Smashwords

6. Google Play Books

Table of Contents

Introduction

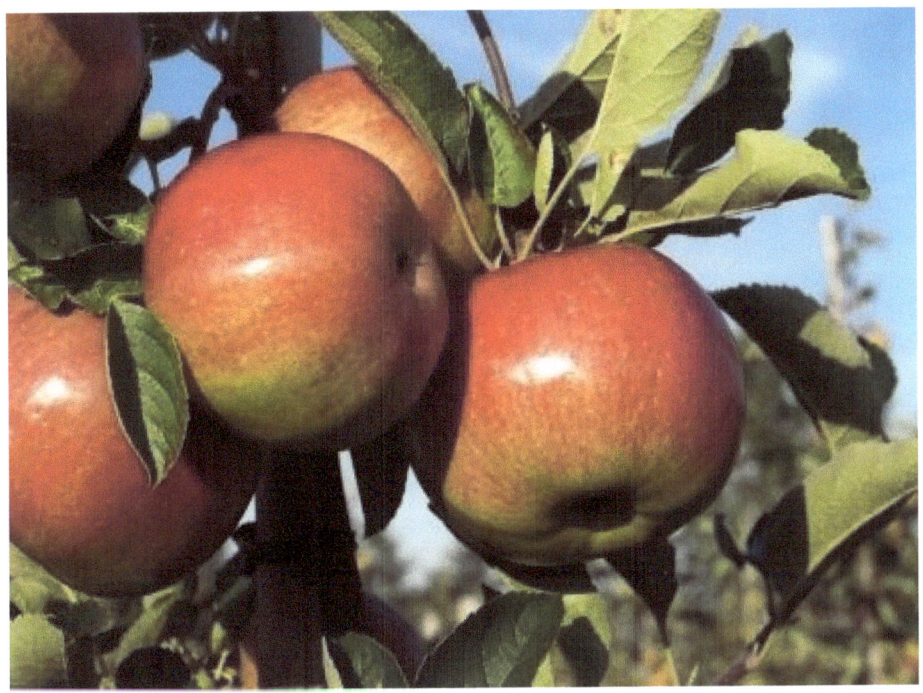

In ancient times, it was said that the Wise men were very careful about their diets. They ate meat very rarely. However, their diet was totally made up of roots, spices, nuts, vegetables and fruit. According to their knowledge, this was the way in which they could ensure good health, absence of diseases and also promote longevity.

Nevertheless, it is a sad thing that in the 21st century, not many of us know how to eat fruit properly. Yes, there is a method of eating fruit in order to gain the proper benefits of fruit. In ancient times, people also knew the rules went to eat fruit in which season and under what circumstances and in which amounts.

That was to prevent people from gorging on fruit. This was a natural reaction, especially when they were extremely hungry and suddenly found themselves confronted with trees and trees of fruit ready to be picked and eaten.

In ancient times, it was said that any fruit which belonged to one particular season had to be eaten in that season itself. That was because nature had made it to benefit the human body, only in that season. That is why seasonal fruits in tropical areas like mangoes, melons, guavas, and cantaloupes grew only in the summer so that they could provide human beings with refreshment as well as plenty of water content which they needed in the summer.

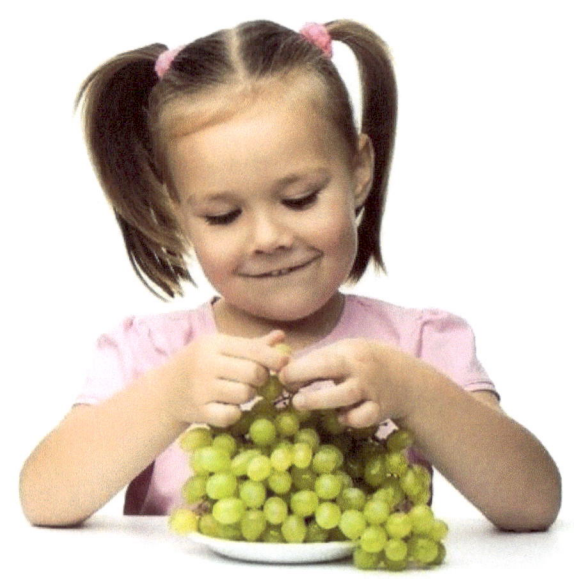

Also, at that time, fruit were never eaten along with meals nor was their juice drunk while you were eating your lunch or dinner. Nevertheless, many of the fruits available in nature to man today are easy to digest. And that is why they were always eaten separately from a regular meal.

That is why here is one point which many of you do not know. When you are having your breakfast, you normally wash it down with fresh fruit juice. I also used to recommend this to people as a healthy addition to the most important meal of the day. Until I found out that fruit juice should be drunk any time in the day, **when you are not eating any meal.**

That is because the time taken to digest the food is different from the time taken to digest fruit juice. So if you want to keep your stomach healthy, allow it to digest food in one go, and at one time and fruit juice or fruit at another time.

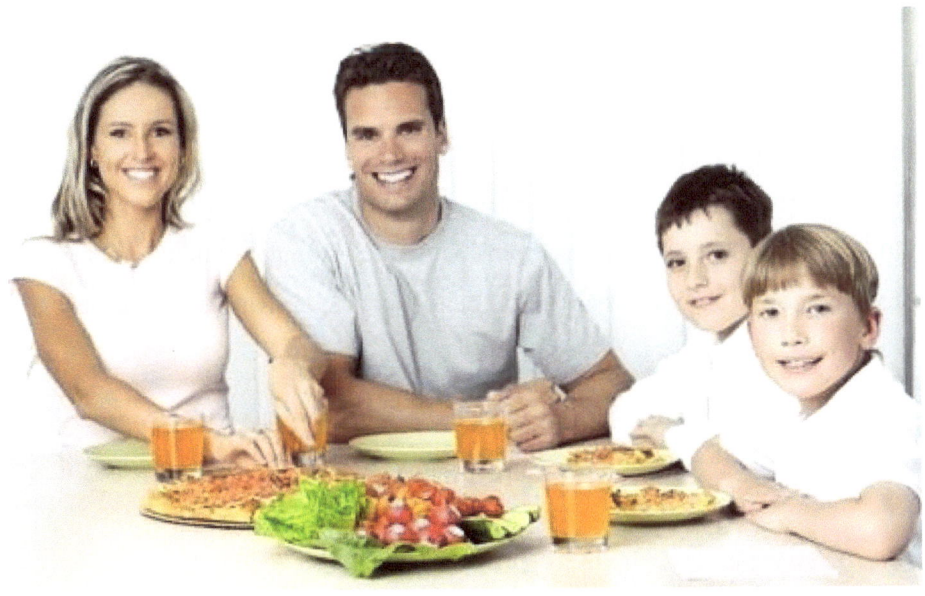

Lots of fruit and vegetables, eaten as salads instead of regular meals are good as starters. Eat your solid/regular meals, 2 hours after you have had fruit juice, raw vegetables and raw fruit. This is going to give your stomach lots of time to digest that fruit juice and nutritional fruit content and to assimilate all its beneficial properties.

The above photograph has a pizza loaded with meat, and other pizza base toppings and with a bread dough base, eaten along with a fruit and vegetable accompaniment and fresh juice. Sorry to say this, but this practice of mixing raw fruits and vegetables along with a heavy meal would have been frowned upon by the ancients!

It is not possible for all fruits to be beneficial to everyone at the same time, because human beings have different physiological and biochemical makeups. Also, they are some fruit, which are not eaten by people suffering from some particular ailments. For example, if you are suffering from asthma or other respiratory problems, nobody told you before not to eat any bananas and guavas. These are definitely not beneficial for people suffering from respiratory problems.

People suffering from diabetes should not eat bananas, grapes, cherries, and mangoes because these have larger quantities of fruit "sugar" in them. And those people who are suffering from "sensitive" stomachs and are more prone to stomach ailments should not eat bananas, guavas, and papayas.

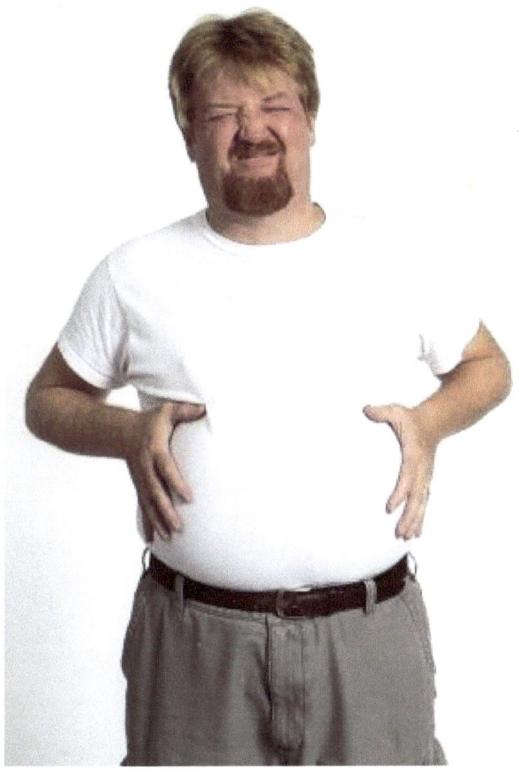

Should not have eaten all those bananas...

He is right. One banana eaten all alone can cause constipation. That is why you have to eat two bananas at a time, accompanied with yogurt in order to keep your stomach healthy. Unless of course you are suffering from asthma and diabetes. That is when you are not going to eat any bananas at all. Though you can eat unsweetened yogurt without any additions of fruit.

Benefiting Tips for Fruit

Many of us are not so lucky as to find fresh fruit right at our doorstep. However fresh and clean fruit are definitely more beneficial than those packed up in packages, and sitting on our supermarket shelves for a couple of days. Any sort of fruit, which has some spots, seems overripe or seems more soft than usual should never be picked or bought.

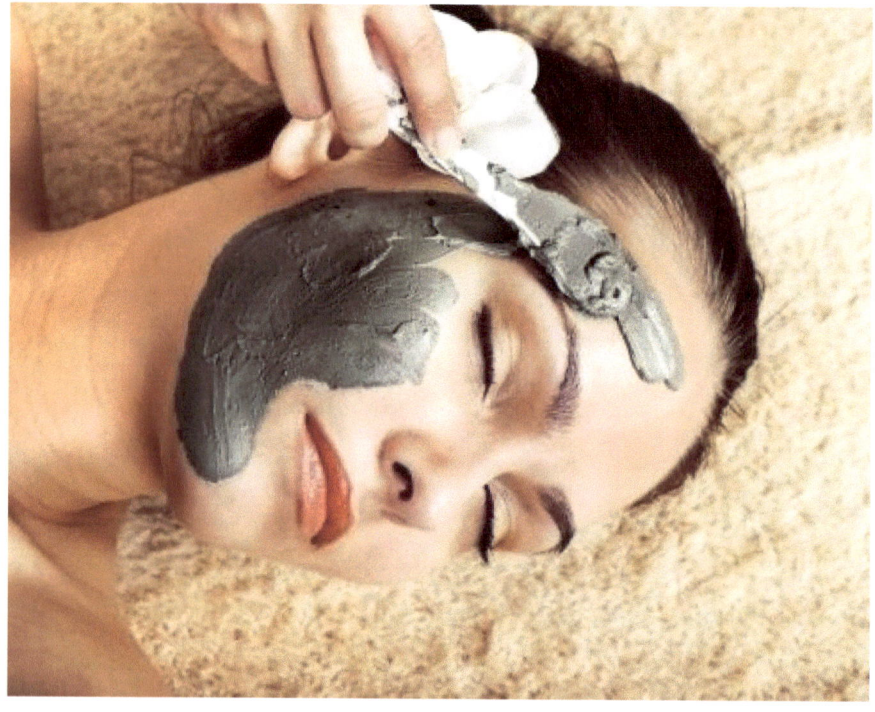

If you are using fruit along with Fuller's Earth in facemasks, make sure that the fruit is fresh and not overripe.

Overripe fruit mean that there nutritional value has started to lessen. Any fruit, which is rotting or has a number of spots or blemishes on it is definitely not good for your health.

I remember a relative of mine who could never be persuaded to eat bananas fresh. Those bananas used to stand on the top of the refrigerator and in a couple of days, the room would start stinking with a fruity smell of overripe bananas. I asked her if she had a prejudice against eating bananas at the right time and what made her prefer bananas with the flesh soggy, smelling over – fruity and definitely not edible.

She immediately said that such banana pulp was exactly right for plastering all over her face in a freshening banana mask, mixed with yogurt and honey! Talk about some mothers having 'em.

When I told her that overripe bananas were not used in facemasks, but the flesh of ripe bananas were, she told me practically that a banana was a banana was a banana.

I saw that same relative after 7 years and she was still complaining how the blemishes on her face could not be removed, even though she kept using facemasks every day. No comment.

Fruit in Its Natural State

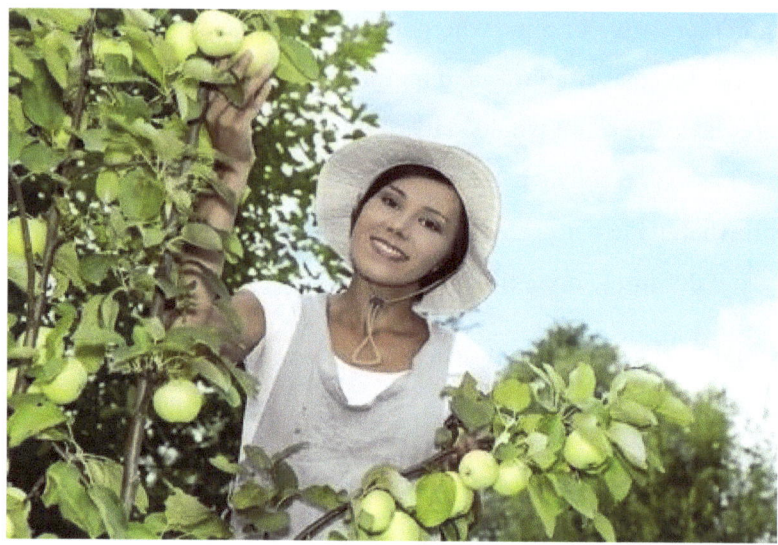

Eat fruit in its natural state. Now this is another thing that most of us do not follow because the moment we pick up a fruit salad, we are going to sprinkle lots of spices, garlic salt, lemon juice and other additives in order to make it more tasty. This counteracts the natural beneficial ingredients present in fruit.

This means that you are going to eat mangoes, grapes, pineapples, melons, cantaloupes, and other juicy fruit without any additives sprinkled on them.

However, natural fruit remedies which are prescribed to cure different types of ailments are normally done with fruit items to which salt, pepper and lemon juice as well as other curative herbs and spices are added. That means you are not eating fruit here for the fun of it. You are eating those spices and fruit mixture as a medical natural curative.

Also, in many fruits, the majority of the nutritional ingredients are present under the surface of the skin. These include apples, pears, guavas, peaches and bananas.

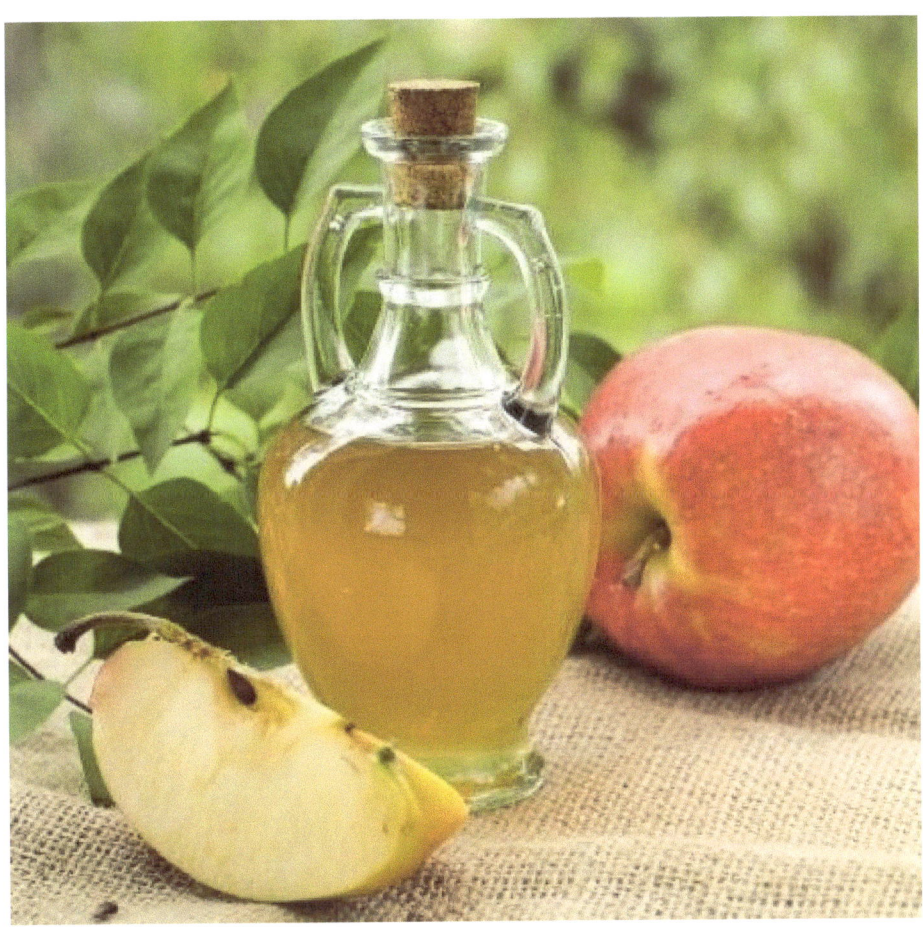

So when you are eating apples, peaches and pears do not peel them, but eat them along with the peels. Some people say that Apple peels are capable of giving them stomach – aches. They will, if you do not masticate the apples well before swallowing.

When I was talking about the nutritional vitamins and minerals present underneath a banana skin, naturally, you would not eat the skin of a banana would you? But you could eat the white portion when you turn over the banana skin. It is normally disregarded because people do not want to be seen scraping the creamy white portion underneath the skin. Try it out.

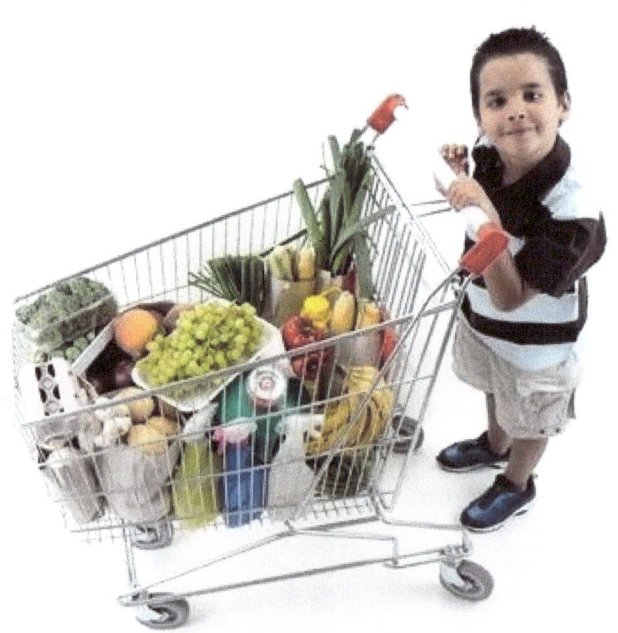

Fruit juice has to be taken out fresh and drunk immediately. I had a couple of colleagues once upon a time, who used to bring fresh fruit juice to the office, and drink it throughout the day. By midafternoon, they would be making faces that the orange juice had turned bitter and there was something wrong with the quality of the oranges they had bought.

When I told them that orange juice was best drunk fresh because it would turn bitter on keeping, they called me a durned interfering Know It All, but that is the truth. Fresh juices begin to turn bitter with the passing of time. Especially when you have mixed up two fruit juices together, like grapes with orange juice. I would not suggest that!

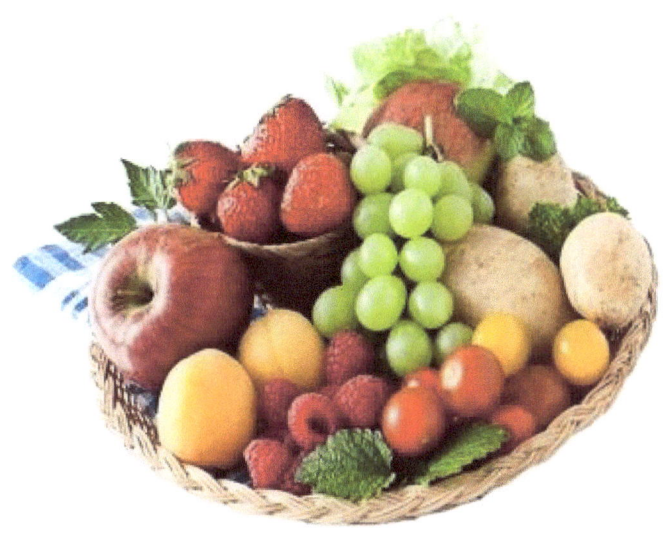

Eat these fruit raw as often as possible without any additives on them.

Detoxification Diet

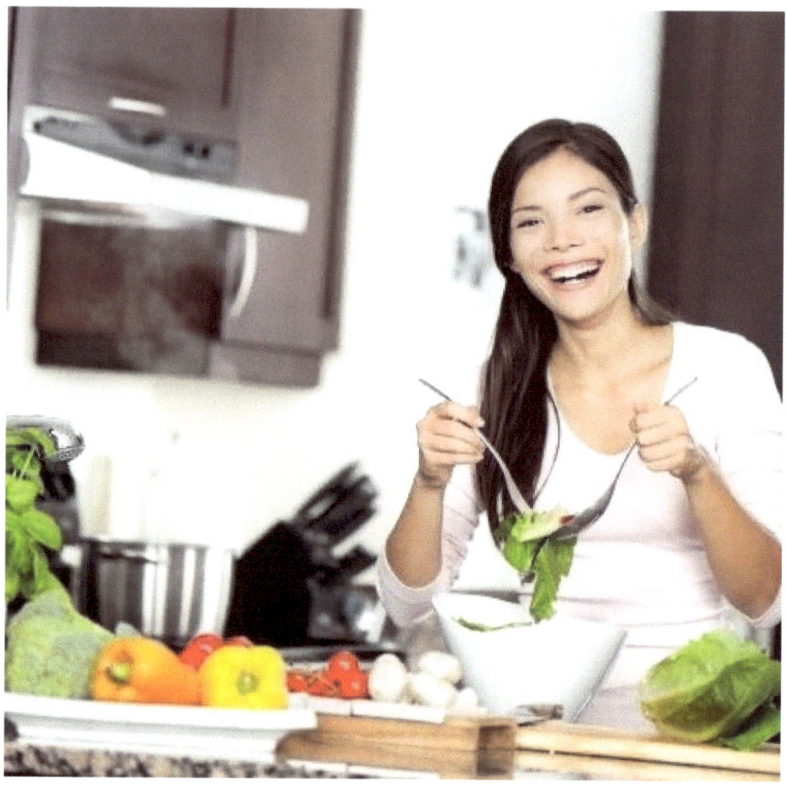

Vegetables can also be included in your detoxification diet as long as they are fresh and raw.

A complete fruit detoxification diet was normally taken by the ancients every week. That was when one day was given over to the eating of fruit and nothing but fruit. This cleared out the system wonderfully well.

Even today, in many parts of the East, there is a detoxification ritual done twice a year which has been inculcated in ancient religious tradition. This is when only fruit, and some special cereals are eaten for 10 days in order to get rid of the toxins. Though naturally, that person is happy doing a religious "fast" for his own spiritual benefit.

I must give it to the ancients. They were an admirable people and really knew how best mankind could be served by putting these natural detoxification methods under the protective mantle of spiritual upliftment and religious tradition.

If they called it detoxification and asked human beings to do it as a general rule, nobody would have bothered to follow it because it was such a bore. On the other hand, it has been followed down the ages, because it is a part of a cultural, religious, and conventional tradition. And that is the reason why this detoxification is done by millions, every year, cleansing heart, body, mind and soul at the same time.

In fact, the body needs detoxification twice a year, and it is done regularly every year. No wonder the ancients were so healthy.

Fruit as Food Substitution

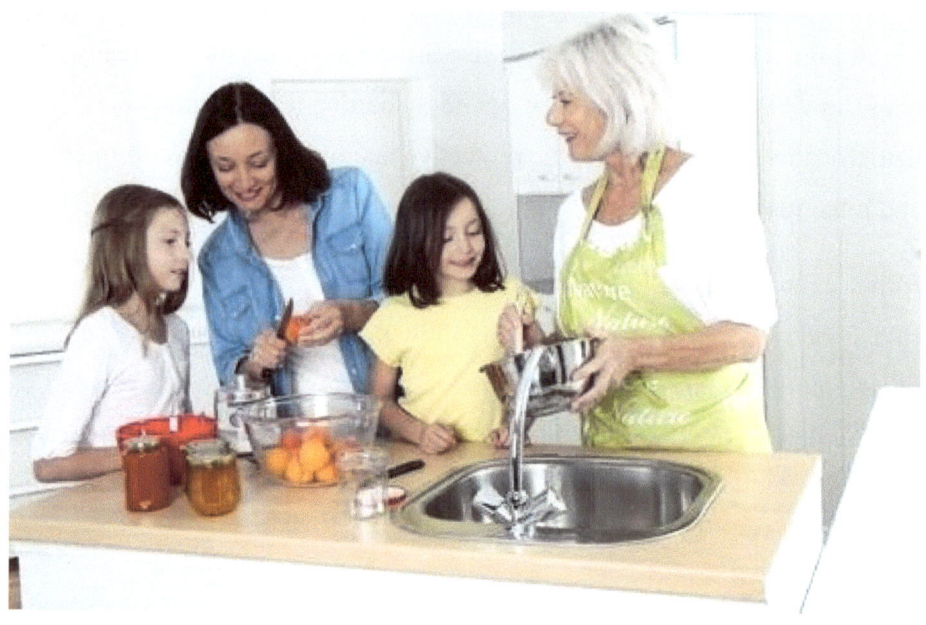

Do not use fruit as a substitute for food. If you think that you are going to get the supplements and nutrition from fruits and stop eating food, you are making a mistake. Fruits have their own place in the nutritional list, and food has its own special place in your diet.

A number of my colleagues missed their meals because they were so busy slaving away on their desks, that they just took out an apple and crunched it. That was their lunch. You may have seen many of your own friends doing the same thing. A regular meal should not be made up of fruit or fruit juice.

That is because fruit juice is so easily digested that it is assimilated really fast into your system. That is why you are going to feel hungry even after you have drunk lots of fruit juice and if you do not provide your body with proper food, you are starving yourself unknowingly and unconsciously.

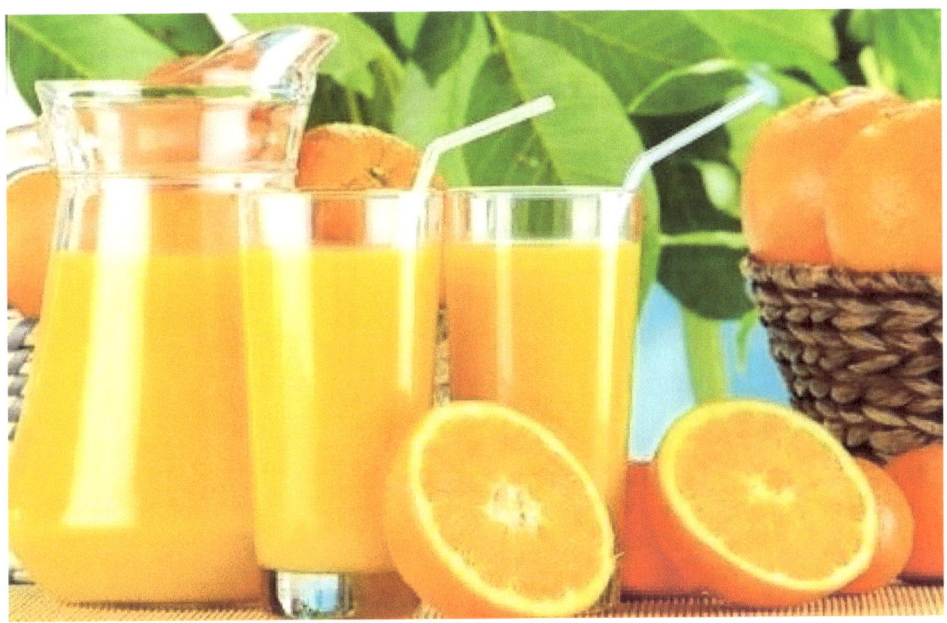

Also, drinking lots of fruit juice is not advisable because it is going to mess up your biochemical physiology. So that means you are not going to drink 8 glasses of fruit juice every day, thinking that it is going to do wonders for your skin. In fact, that much fruit juice content in your body is going to make you unwell later on.

Do not eat raw fruit, even though this could not be taught to us children, when we were kids. We loved plucking raw fruit from the trees, like guavas, mangoes, gooseberries, and whatever came within the range of our vision and chomping on them. And naturally we blamed all the stomachaches to anything and everything else, including Bad water , the tasty lunch we ate, the weather or any other excuse which came in hand or mind.

Fruit is always supposed to be eaten fresh. Do not preserve it in the fridge for a little while, and chill it, before you enjoy a meal of chilled fruit. That is because the moment the cut fruit is left exposed to the open-air it is going to lose its nutritional content and value. All the fruit with a delicate and thin outer cover come in this category.

Also, this is one new thing I learned about fruits. There are some fruit, which are not eaten after dusk. That is because they are comparatively difficult to digest, especially while you are asleep. These include guavas, Popeye as and bananas. These are the fruit which have lots of water included in the pulp. As they take a while to digest, like I said before, avoid eating them at night. The best time to eat fruit is before breakfast.

Healing through Fruit

Here are some common fruits given, which you are going to find easily available in your city. They have some natural time-tested healing powers, which you can implement right now.

Lemons

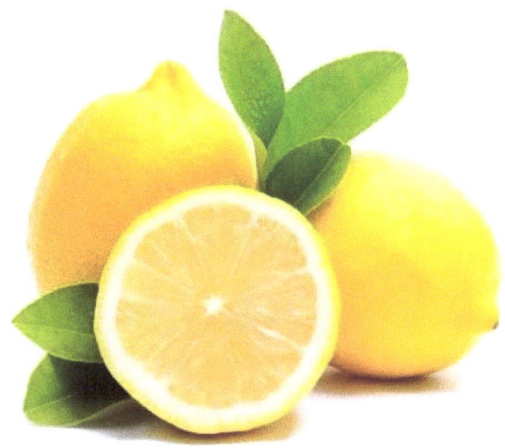

Lemons are an excellent source of vitamin C. They are definitely good for boosting up your immunity system as well as your metabolism. Here are some common ways in which you can get the full benefit of lemons –

As a Pimple Cure

Just take 3 teaspoons full of cream and add 1 tablespoon full of lemon juice in it. Apply this paste upon the affected areas for one month. The lemon juice is a very powerful antibiotic and antiseptic. It is going to get rid of the infection. It is also going to clear up your skin of any blemishes.

Nausea and Giddiness

Lime squash has been a timeworn remedy as a coolant, and a refreshing drink in the summer down the ages. That is the reason why, people drinking lemon juice turned into lemon squash with plenty of ice and sugar on never going to suffer from dehydration, nausea, sunstroke, or giddiness.

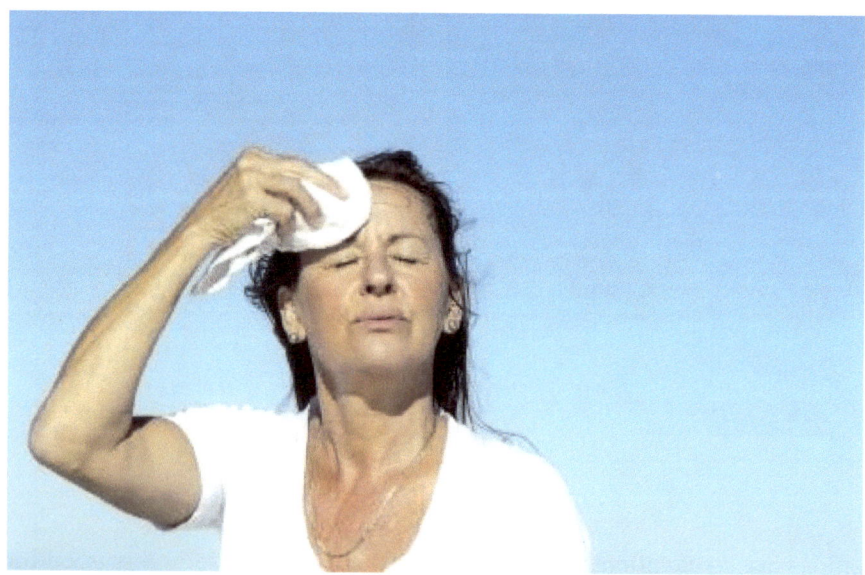

Take half a lemon, and squeeze it in 3 teaspoons full of water. Add a couple of seeds of crushed cardamom seeds to this liquid, and give it to the patient after every 2 hours. This stops any harmful side effects of sunstroke, and gets rid of the giddiness and nausea too.

If you are suffering from giddiness due to flatulence or acidity squeeze a lemon in a cup of hot water, and drink it as often as possible. This is going to get rid of the giddiness as well as the stomach problems. However, if you are suffering from heartburn, just squeeze the lemon in one cup of **cold water**.

Stomachaches

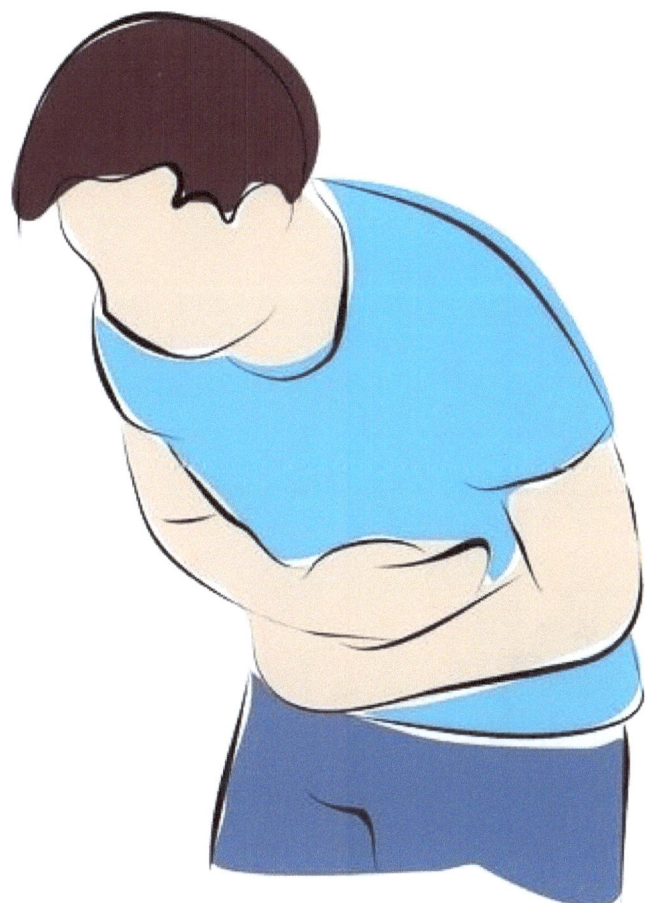

Stomachaches may be caused due to our large number of reasons including overeating and infections caused by viruses and bacteria. This can be prevented as well as cured by taking one teaspoonful each of sugar, bishops weed, cumin seeds and rock salt. Crush them together and put the mixture in a bottle.

Now take half a teaspoonful of this mixture and mix it with a little lemon juice – one quarter of a lemon – and drink it down with hot water. This is going to get rid of your stomachache and any sort of infection. It is also going to aid in digestion, if the stomachache was caused through overeating.

Lemon for Weight Loss

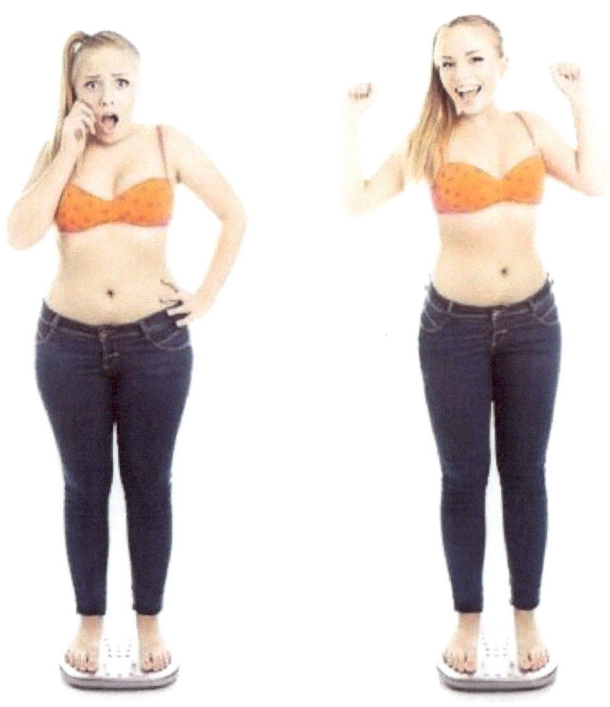

I have seen a number of my friends, drinking lots of lemon juice first thing in the morning, hoping against hope to lose some weight. But they are going about it the wrong way. You need to drink one lemon in 250 g of warm water, first thing in the morning, without even washing out your mouth or eating anything else. This has to be done only in the summer not in any other time of the year. Two months of doing this is going to lessen your weight in a systematic fashion.

Bananas

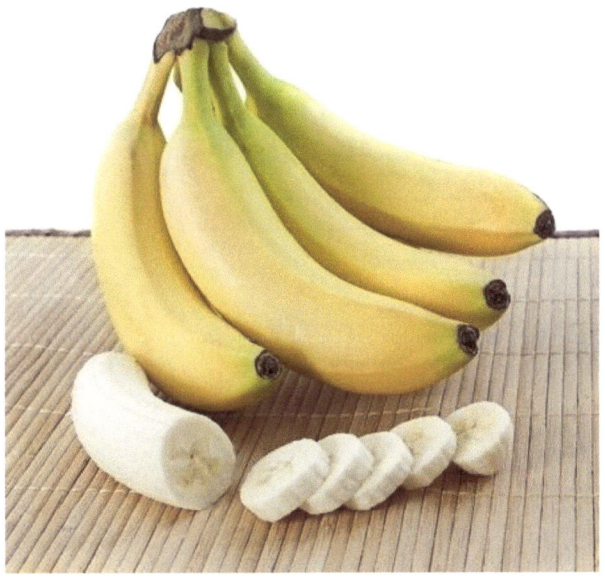

Bananas are a powerhouse of carbohydrates. Eat them regularly and you are going to have a glowing skin, and a healthy body.

Angina

People suffering from angina have to be very careful about their lifestyle. Apart from their drugs, recommended to them by their doctors, they have to have something which keeps them healthy and prevents any possible chance of a heart attack. This is done by eating 2 bananas in 2 tablespoons full of honey every morning, one are before you have your breakfast.

Bananas for Weight Gain

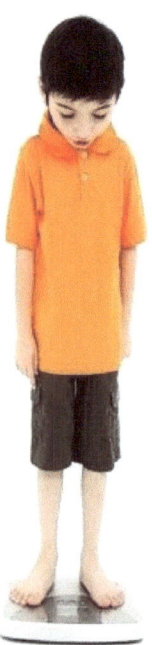

There are some people who want to gain some weight. This was my case. As the grass was always greener on the other side of the fence, I hated my skeletal thin, lanky, and uncoordinated awkward self when I was at college. I looked at the full and one could almost say voluptuous mother earth goddess figures of most of my friends and envied them. Almost 3 decades later, all these ladies are very obese and have a definite weight problem.

But at that time I wanted to be plump and that is why a helper in our university hostel who was an herbalist told me this natural remedy to put on weight. This is time-tested.

Eat 2 bananas with a glassful of hot milk everyday for 2 months. You are definitely going to find yourself putting on weight. However, if you suffer from flatulence, do not eat this remedy.

Incidentally, that "white witch" was responsible for making up an herbal remedy to make my hair grow again. Childhood illnesses had made me suffer from alopecia due to a vitamin B deficiency. So the bald patches, which are definitely not very common in females made me feel really embarrassed until she told me that she would make up a cure for me. She did.

I had a 400 g tin of this wonderful natural cure which was a brown grease like paste. I applied it for 15 days on all the patches, and they disappeared, never to come back again.

Unfortunately I was not sensible enough at that time to take down that recipe which would have made me a billionaire because the healthy hair growth has not stopped to this day, and there is absolutely no question of any alopecia. This much I knew that she had added some natural herbs to clarified butter. I could smell the strong aroma of that butter.

Ten years later, I decided that I needed that recipe, like right now because age had brought sense and went back to that city. Nobody knew where she was. So I came back disappointed and for the last 30 years I have been trying to find out that natural remedy for curing baldness permanently.

Anyway, here is another recipe for baldness which I managed to find, when I was hunting for the original long-lost recipe. It is rather tiresome, but if you are not suffering from genetic and inherited baldness, you are going to find your hair growing within a couple of months.

Take out the pulp of an Armenian cucumber. This is not the ordinary cucumber, which we normally eat in salads. This is the slimmer and more delicate version of the normal sturdy cucumber. Anyway, apply the pulp on the affected regions for about a week or so, and you are going to see the hair begin to grow again. Continue this until you have your required hair growth and all the bald patches are sprouting hair there and everywhere.

However, if the hair follicles have been destroyed through heat, exposure to the sun or if you are genetically prone to baldness, this is not going to work for you.

Acidity

In the same way, cucumbers as well as these Armenian cucumbers are quite efficient in getting rid of acidity in your stomach. All you have to do is eat them without adding any salt. However, if you eat them with salt, the moment you eat something else, after that salty mouthful, those things are going to cause acidity in your stomach! Interesting is not it.

Also, remember not to drink any water after you have eaten cucumbers Armenian cucumbers. I saw a friend of mine not drinking any water after her meals, but eating cucumbers. She says that this is a very healthy option and I must agree with her. These cucumbers can be eaten along with your meal as long as you do not sprinkle lots of salt on them.[1] This is a well-known time-tested remedy coming down the ages and which are being used even today.

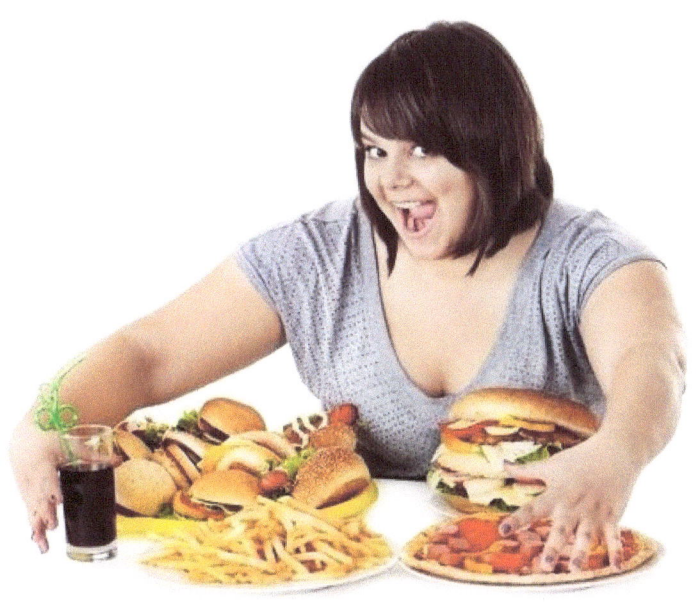

Food eaten in such large quantities is going to cause acidity…

Bananas for Stomach Ailments

If you are suffering from persistent stomach problems, just try eating 2 bananas in a bowl full of yogurt everyday. This is going to take care of

---

[1] So now I know the reason why I suffered from acidity whenever I ate a cucumber salad with lots of salt, pepper and lemon sprinkled on it, and I have been blaming the spicy and roasted chicken for that, all the while.

cramps, stomach disorders, and other ailments caused through overeating or an impaired digestive system.

Pineapples

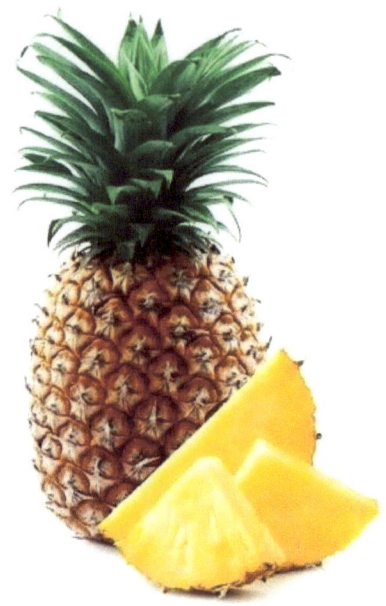

Pineapples may have been considered exotic 50 years ago, but thanks to the world, getting smaller, we are able to get pineapples in our respective cities in all corners of the globe quite frequently.

Dyspepsia

Pineapples are the only fruit, which is eaten with a mixture of black pepper and rock salt in order to get rid of flatulence and dyspepsia. Peel them fresh and mix them with black pepper and rock salt.

Edema

Edema is normally caused by a number of reasons, which includes hot weather, dehydration, and even a mild heart problem. By the time you reach your 40s, you may find yourself suffering from a swelling in your feet, especially after you have spent the whole day either standing on them or sitting on them.

If you are suffering from edema, include a whole pineapple in your diet chart for the day. 10 days and you are going to see a great reduction in the swelling. 20 days, and you are going to see your feet as thin and slim as they were when you were 20. This pineapple intake hydrates your body, and gets rid of the toxins. It also provides your body with supporting nutrients so there is absolutely going to be no swelling in any part of your body.

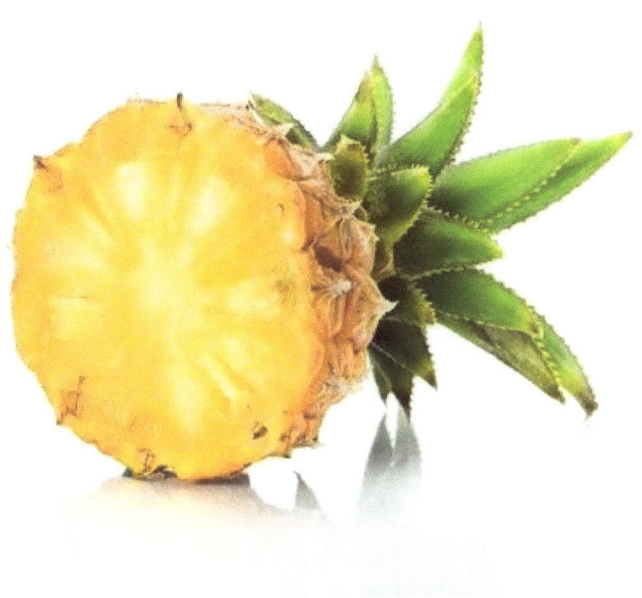

Incontinence

If you continue eating pineapples, freshly cut throughout your life, you are not going to suffer from incontinence ever. And if you suffer from frequent urination, just cut up some pineapple pieces and juice them. Mix the juice with a small quantity of powdered cumin seeds, powdered nutmeg and black salt. This mixture drunk morning and evening is going to get rid of any sort of infection in your stomach, causing frequent urination.

Grapes

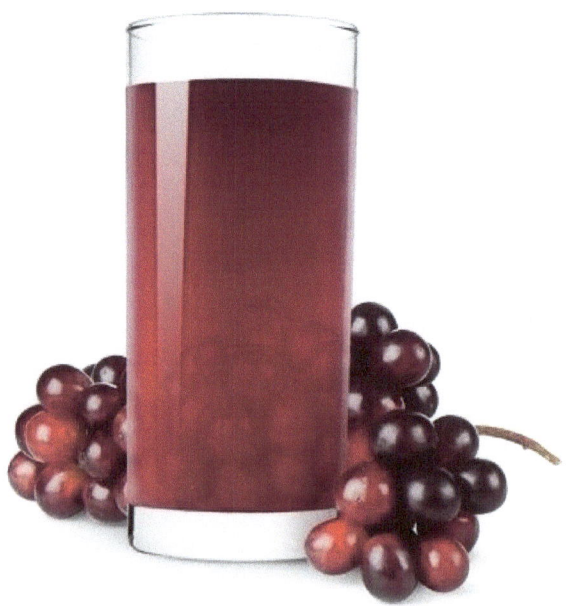

Since ancient times, grapes have been considered to be the food of the gods and their gift given to mankind, because of their many beneficial properties. Grape juice was drunk in such large quantities every day, fermented and unfermented that they never suffered from tumors, cancer, and toxin buildup.

Since ancient times, 50 g of fresh grape juice prevented people suffering from digestive problems, dyspepsia, constipation, headaches, giddiness and flatulence.

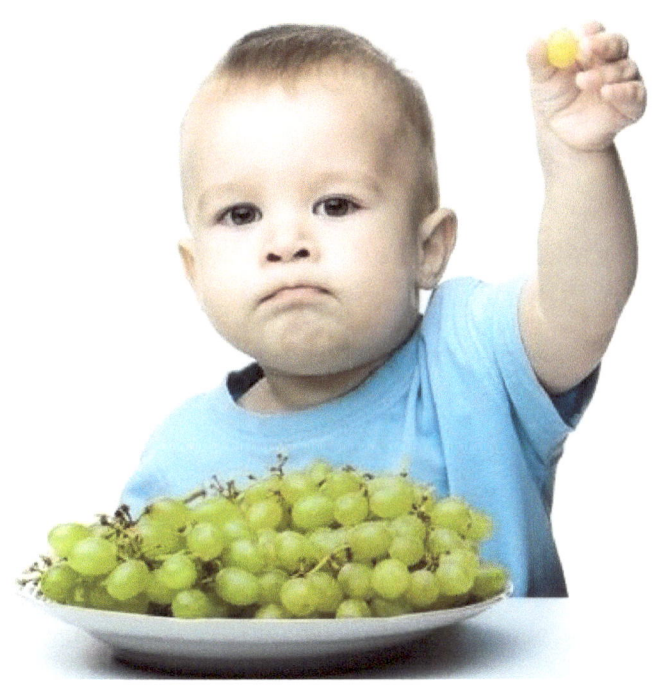

Epilepsy Cure

Here is an ancient remedy for epilepsy which may not be acknowledged by people in the West because they have not researched much in the healing powers of an herb called akarkara.[2] [Anacyclus pyrethrum.] It is an indigenous herb only found in the Indian subcontinent and that is why it has been used in ancient herbal treatises down the ages.

To get rid of epilepsy, you will need to grind 10 g of this plant's root with 20 g of deseeded black raisins. Put them in half a cup full of water, and boil to make a decoction. Infuse for 10 minutes, off the heat and place it in a glass bottle.

Now you are going to take less than a quarter teaspoon of this very powerful mixture [2 g.] with milk every day. This prevents epileptic fits. It also slowly cures epilepsy.

Dry Cough

Dry cough normally occurs when you are suffering from an irritation in the throat passage. For this all you need is 10 g of crushed almonds, 10 g of licorice root and 10 g of deseeded raisins. Mix them all together, and make into small pea-sized pellets with the help of a little bit of water. Suck two pellets 4 times a day, like you would do a piece of rock candy, until you get rid of the dry cough within a couple of days.

You can also get rid of the dry cough by taking 20 g of ripe pomegranate skin, sun-dried and powdered and mix it with 4 g of rock salt. Add a little bit of water and make pea-sized pellets of about 1 g each. Suck two pellets 4 times a day, until the dry cough disappears. Do not eat anything sour during this curing time.

---

[2] https://www.ayurtimes.com/anacyclus-pyrethrum-akarkara-benefits-uses-side-effects/

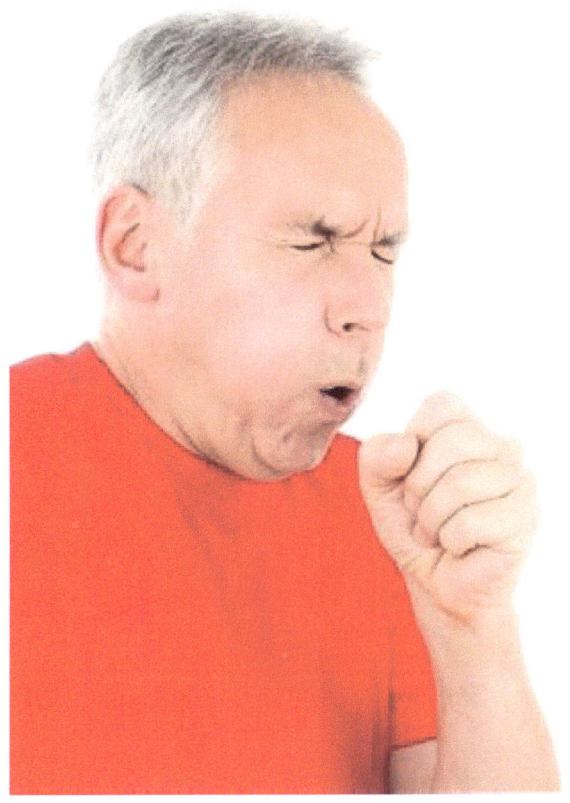

Lung Infections

These normally take place in the winter, when the body is vulnerable to infections. To cure this, the ancients put 10 almonds and 10 black raisins in water overnight. The next morning, they de-skinned the almonds and deseeded the raisins. After that they took a little piece of ginger and ground all 3 of them together into a smooth paste. This was mixed with 2 tablespoons full of honey and fed to the patient twice a day.

This gives strength to the lungs and prevented any sort of infections there, including emphysema. Naturally, the patient was not allowed to smoke at all, because that causes emphysema.

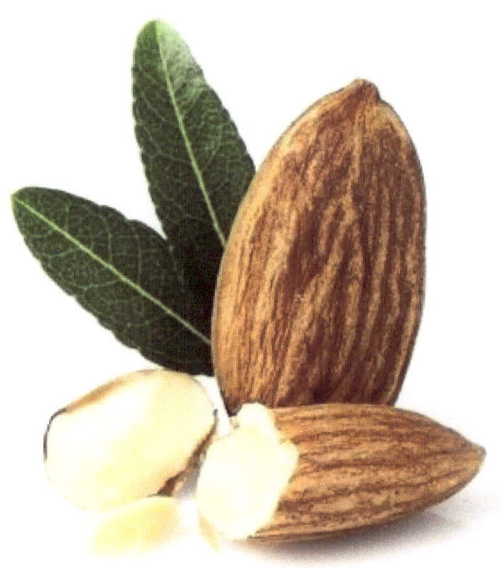

One of my Army friends was going on a posting to the mountainous high-altitude areas, and asked me to give his wife this recipe to keep the whole family healthy in the cold weather where body resistance is low and chances of lung infection is high. I told him to take a couple of bottles of pure honey from down here in the plains and lots of dry fruit, including almonds, because the children loved them, especially in the winter. I also told him that it would not harm him any if he added a little bit of other dry fruits like raisins, powdered walnuts and pistachios to the mixture. He obeyed with alacrity!

I also gave this remedy to a friend in Montana, who suffered a lot during the Montana blizzards! She said that it was very effective. But the only problem was that she really hated ginger! Unfortunately ginger is necessary in this cure, because it keeps your system healthy. But I told her to boost up the amount of honey with half a teaspoonful more. She is not complaining any now!

Boils and Carbuncles

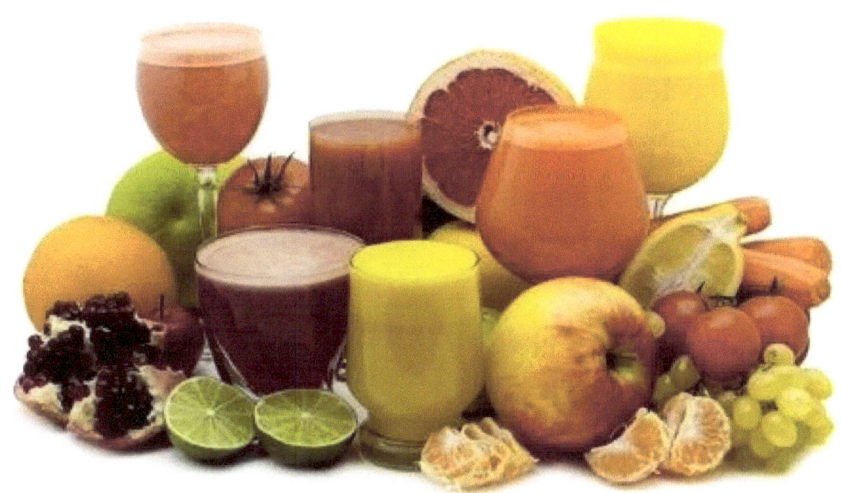

Boils and carbuncles were once upon a time a way of life because people did not bother much about hygienic surroundings and infections then. That was the reason why skin interrupted into infections which would begin to show suppuration and infection, if it was not treated properly. So in ancient times, all one had to do is make a paste of a little bit of deseeded raisins, some aloe vera pulp, a little bit of honey and some crushed basil leaves or some fresh green neem leaves if you had them around.

This was placed on the carbuncle or on the boil, before you went to bed. It was then covered with a piece of cloth and left to cure itself. The bandage was opened up in the morning and refreshed again until all the infection was drawn away.

Apples

One is getting tired of that old cliché telling us that an Apple a day keeps the doctor away. But there is some justification here because apples are very rich in vitamin B and vitamin C. That is why they keep your mind and body healthy.

Chronic Headaches

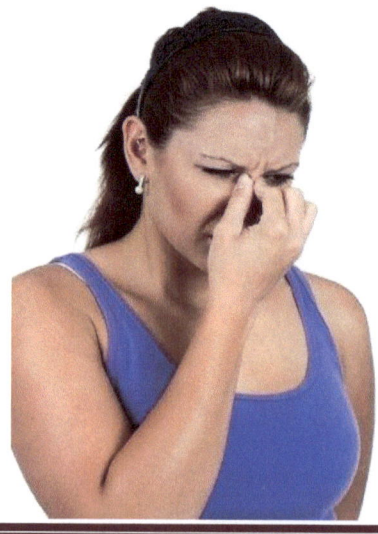

If you are suffering from chronic headaches or even tension headaches, all you have to do is pick up a ripe sweet juicy apple. Eat it on an empty stomach with salt 1st thing in the morning. Do this for 15 days and your chronic headaches will have gone, never to reappear back again.

Excessive Thirst

In the same manner, if you are suffering from excessive thirst and a dry mouth, even though you keep drinking lots of water, all you have to do is take 30 g of apple juice in 30 g of water. Drink this once a day for a couple of days and you are going to see your mouth not feeling dry at all or you feeling thirsty excessively.

Mental Fatigue

People normally suffer from mental fatigue brought about by stress and tension. You feel that you cannot concentrate anymore, and find yourself trying to remember things which needed to be done, and you are still trying to make out how to do them and went to do them and why to do them. Been there, borne that.

To get your mental concentration levels back again to normal, eat one ripe sweet apple along with its skin, 10 minutes before you have your meals. Do this at lunch and dinner. However, you are not going to eat any rice, potatoes or any spicy food when you are undergoing this natural cure. Do this for 10 days and find yourself feeling mentally and physically fit, yet once again.

Pomegranates

Pomegranates once came in the category of exotic fruit, normally found in tropical regions. They were considered to be delicacies in Europe over a long period of time until the late 19th century when transportation methods began to improve. So that is why now, pomegranates can be used for natural remedies all over the world through ancient medical recipes taken from China, and in the Middle East.

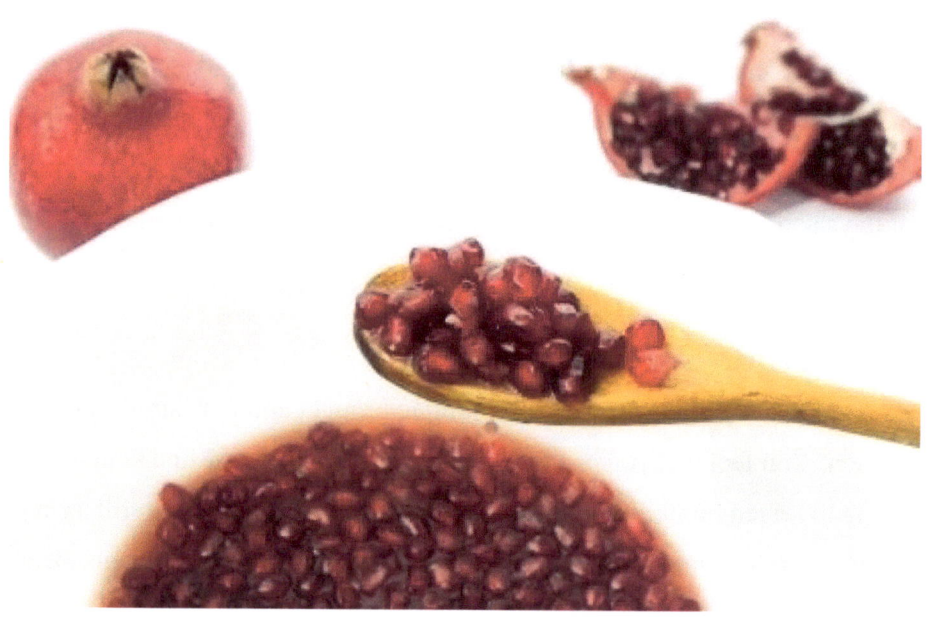

Pomegranates for Your Teeth

It was in Persia that the flower of the pomegranate began to be considered as the symbolic epitome of feminine beauty. Calling a dainty maiden a "pomegranate bud" meant that she was of the quality of which poets would write verses. And this beauty was supported with white, healthy, and clean teeth. So that beauty's grandmother made sure that her granddaughter cleaned her teeth with a paste of powdered pomegranate skin dried in the sun, mixed with salt, every day without fail.

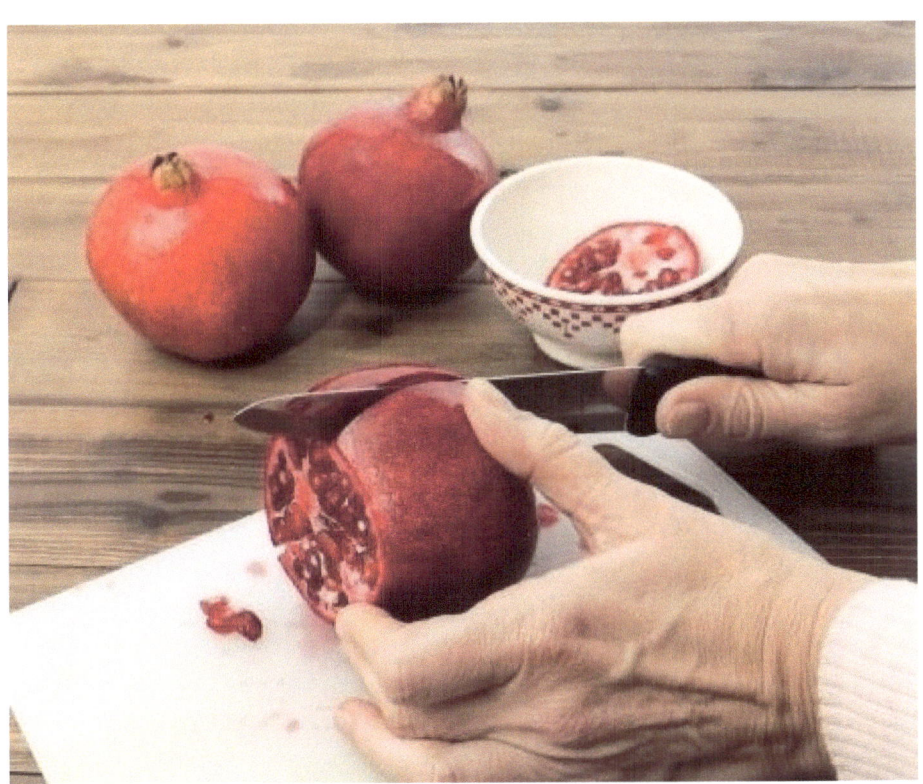

So that was for the teeth. The gums were kept healthy with the addition of powdered sun – dried pomegranate flowers in the above toothpaste mixture. This also prevented bad breath, bleeding of the gums, and gingivitis.

Urinary Infections

Urinary infections are so common today that we immediately go to the doctor and take the prescribed antibiotics given to us. What we do not know is that those antibiotics are getting rid of the infection temporarily. However, the main source of the infection is still present in the body just waiting for a chance to make its appearance again.

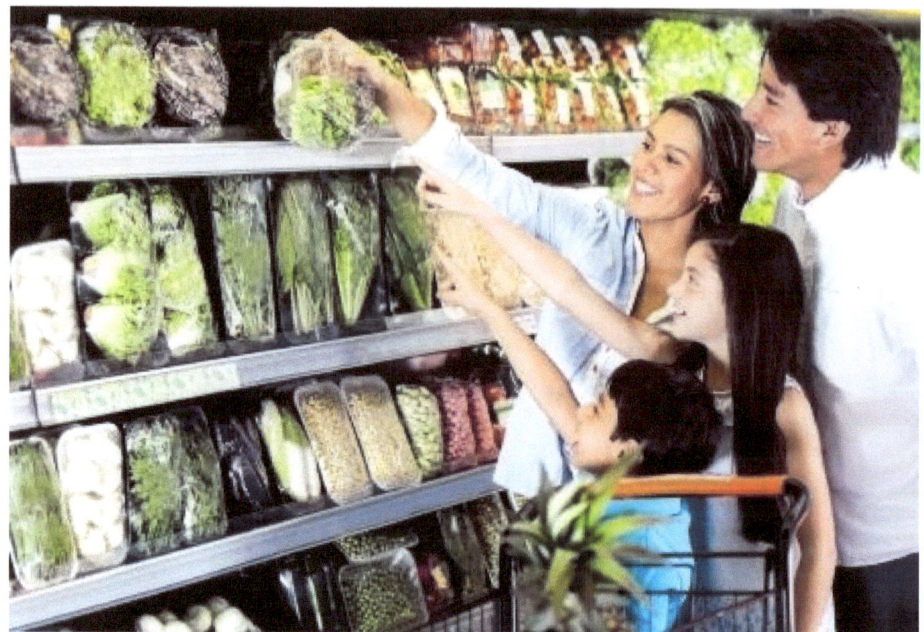

Plenty of fresh fruit and vegetables are going to keep your system free of any sort of infections.

So if you are suffering from continuous or intermittent urinary infections, you may want to cleanse your system from inside with orange juice, pineapple juice, or any other fresh juice at least twice a day.

Along with that, you are going to take 4 g of sun dried pomegranate skin and put it in a glassful of fresh water. Drink this twice a day. This is going to get rid of your urinary infections within 10 days. Do not eat any rice in the meanwhile.

Jaundice

Jaundice has been treated down the ages with the help of pomegranate seeds. Take 50 g of sweet ripe pomegranate seeds and extract the juice. Place the juice in an iron pot. You may ask why an iron pot, but this is the way the ancients treated their patients. They felt that jaundice was caused by an iron and other minerals deficiency, and that juice was left overnight.

The next morning you added crystalline rock sugar/candy according to your taste to this mixture and drank it down. Jaundice would be cured within 20 – 25 days of this treatment. The patient was not given anything sour and spicy to eat during this treatment.

Now remember that all these treatments were done in times when nobody knew about state-of-the-art medical technology and antibiotics and medicines. They used herbal remedies to cure diseases and this was the way in which they treated jaundice down the ages. They also gave the patient lots of fresh sugar cane juice, to help him grow back healthy.

I remember as a child, my younger brother suffering from a mild case of jaundice. He was immediately put on a lot of antibiotics and my grandmother fed him with   boiled food without any spice or fat. The neighbors who had their own advice to give asked her to give him plenty of sugarcane juice. He was cured within the month, though I am not really sure whether it was the boiled food without the spice or the sugarcane juice which cured him. As far as I am concerned, the antibiotics were just for show, with their own side effects for which he had to take other medicines to get rid of those side effects. Until one fine day, father said that he had enough and threw the medicines out. According to him lots of healthy fresh food, fresh air, lots of exercise and no tension about his health would restore my brother back to his state of good health. It did.

Conclusion

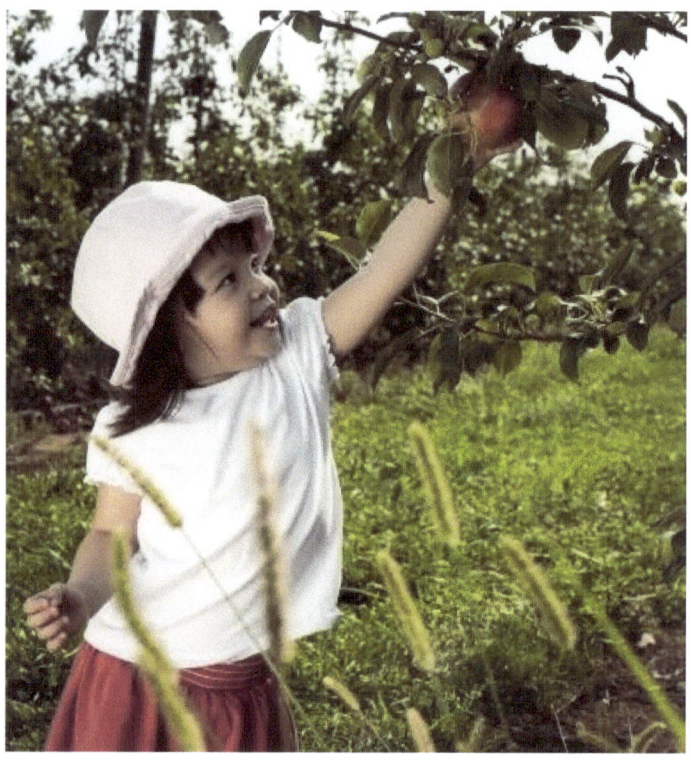

This book has given you a lot of tips, especially time-tested ones, to help you stay healthy with the eating of lots of fruit, fresh and ripe. I am giving you some tips for vegetables, which are time-tested, and are useful even today.

In ancient times, when we did not have stainless steel and other utensils in which to cook our food, this food was normally cooked in copper or alloy metal utensils, if clay pots were not available. So if you have the habit of using grandma's copper or cast-iron vessels to cook vegetables, please cease, desist. They should be cooked in steel vessels as far as possible.

Here is one tip told to me by a friend. If you want to keep green vegetables for a long time, wrap them in some air proof **damp** paper and put them in your fridge. Do not use print paper. Do not use damp cloth vegetable bags, because that is going to rot the vegetables. You can also place them in an air tight polythene paper in the topmost shelf of your fridge.

Make sure that you keep watching these plastic bags often, to see if there is any moisture collection on the sides of the bags. If that is so, take out the bags, and wipe the moisture clean with a dry cloth. If the moisture is left in that bag, it is going to rot your vegetables.

Wash these vegetables only once, before you cut them. Many of us have this habit of washing the vegetables before we refrigerate them. Washing them again and again is going to remove many of the nutritional ingredients present in the vegetables. You may want to dust them properly before you refrigerate them or just wipe them clean with a dry cloth. Washing is going to be done when you take them out before cutting and cooking.

If you have a problem with boiling potatoes, and find that they may look all boiled from outside, but are still raw from the inside, easy, just add a little bit of lemon juice and a pinch of sugar to the water before boiling. Your potatoes are going to get boiled perfectly. In the same manner, you can preserve the color of the boiling vegetables like when you are boiling peas, by adding one fourth teaspoonful of salt to the water before putting it to the boil.

Stay Healthy, Live Long and Prosper!

Author Bio

Dueep Jyot Singh is a Management and IT Professional who managed to gather Postgraduate qualifications in Management and English and Degrees in Science, French and Education while pursuing different enjoyable career options like being an hospital administrator, IT,SEO and HRD Database Manager/ trainer, movie , radio and TV scriptwriter, theatre artiste and public speaker, lecturer in French, Marketing and Advertising, ex-Editor of Hearts On Fire (now known as Solstice) Books Missouri USA, advice columnist and cartoonist, publisher and Aviation School trainer, ex-moderator on Medico.in, banker, student councilor ,travelogue writer … among other things!

One fine morning, she decided that she had enough of killing herself by Degrees and went back to her first love -- writing. It's more enjoyable! She already has 48 published academic and 14 fiction- in- different- genre books under her belt.

When she is not designing websites or making Graphic design illustrations for clients , she is browsing through old bookshops hunting for treasures, of which she has an enviable collection – including R.L. Stevenson, O.Henry, Dornford Yates, Maurice Walsh, De Maupassant, Victor Hugo, Sapper, C.N. Williamson, "Bartimeus" and the crown of her collection- Dickens "The Old Curiosity Shop," and "Martin Chuzzlewit" and so on… Just call her "Renaissance Woman") - collecting herbal remedies, acting like Universal Helping Hand/Agony Aunt, or escaping to her dear mountains for a bit of exploring, collecting herbs and plants, and trekking.

Check out some of the other JD-Biz Publishing books

Gardening Series on Amazon

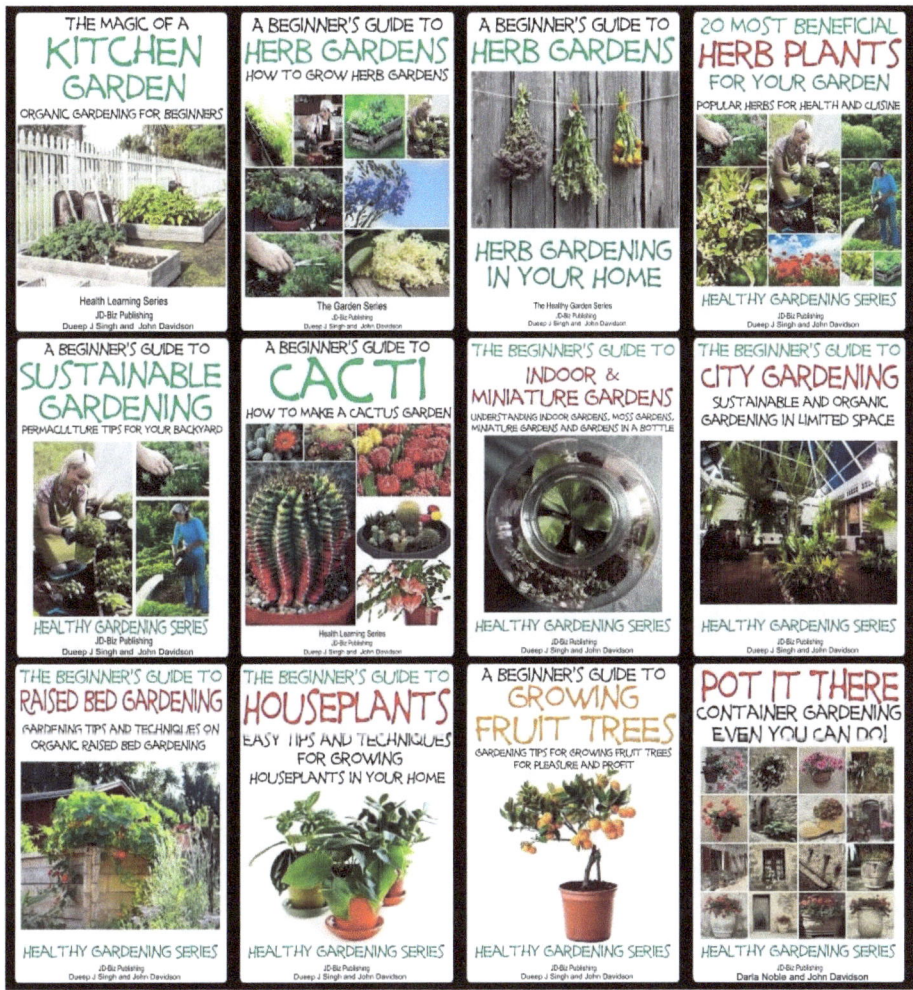

Download Free Books!

http://MendonCottageBooks.com

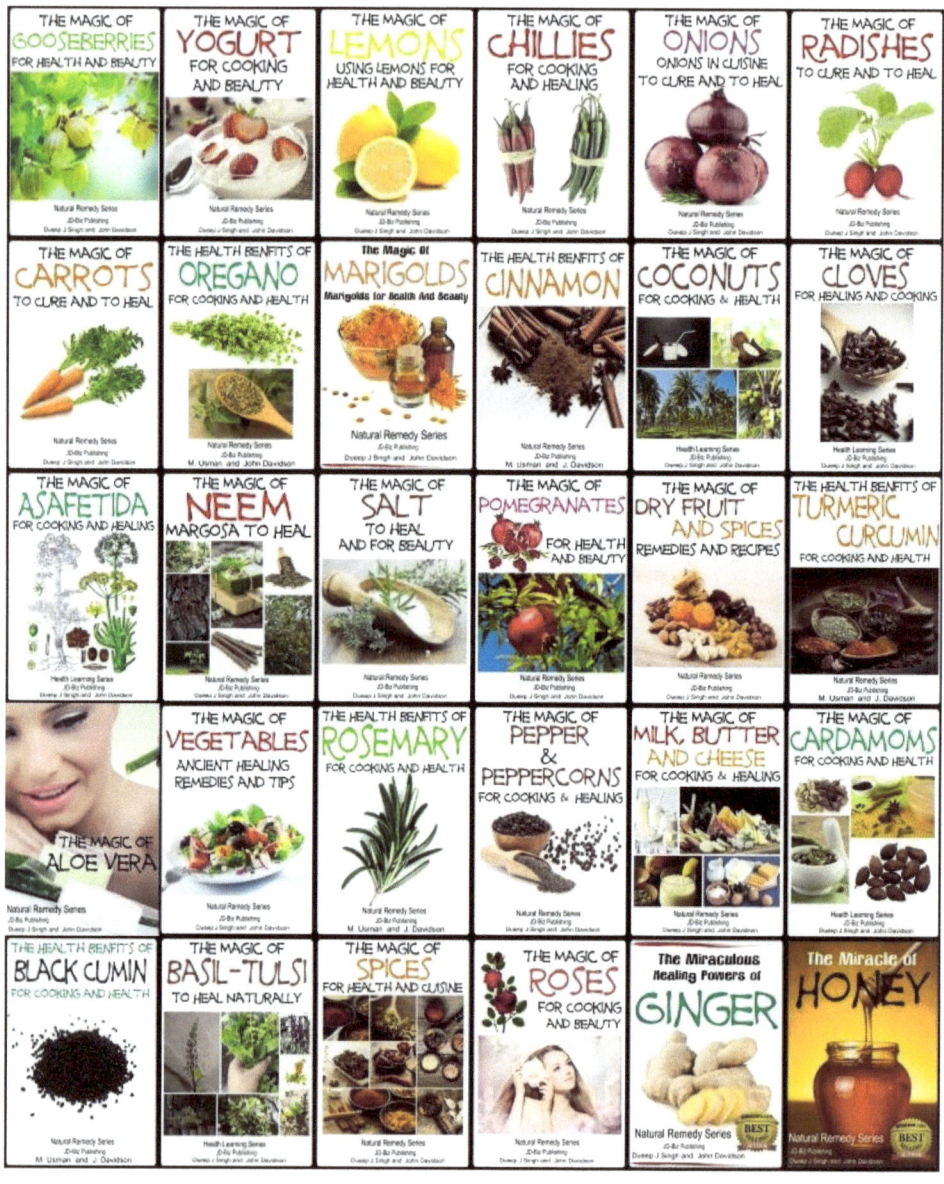

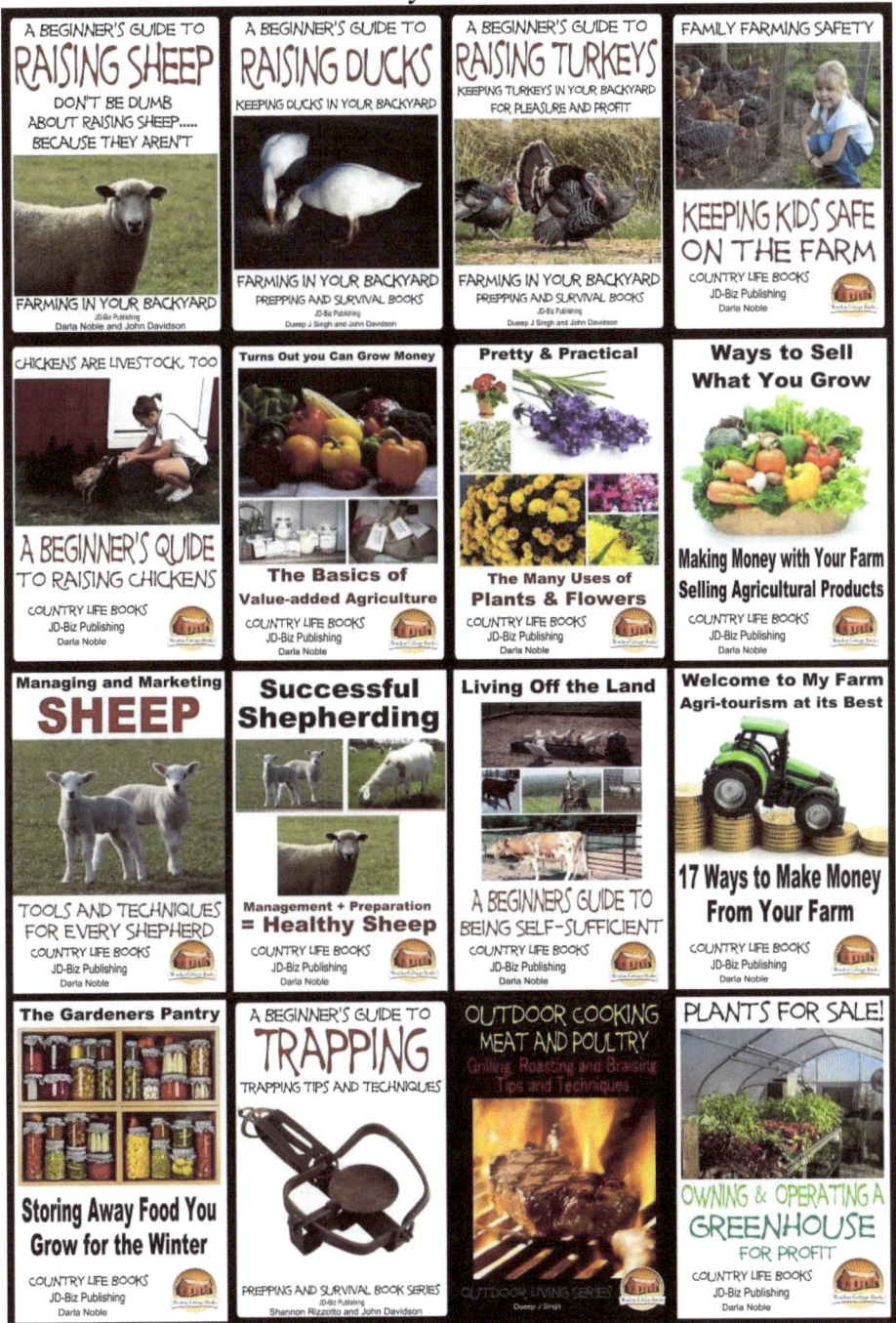

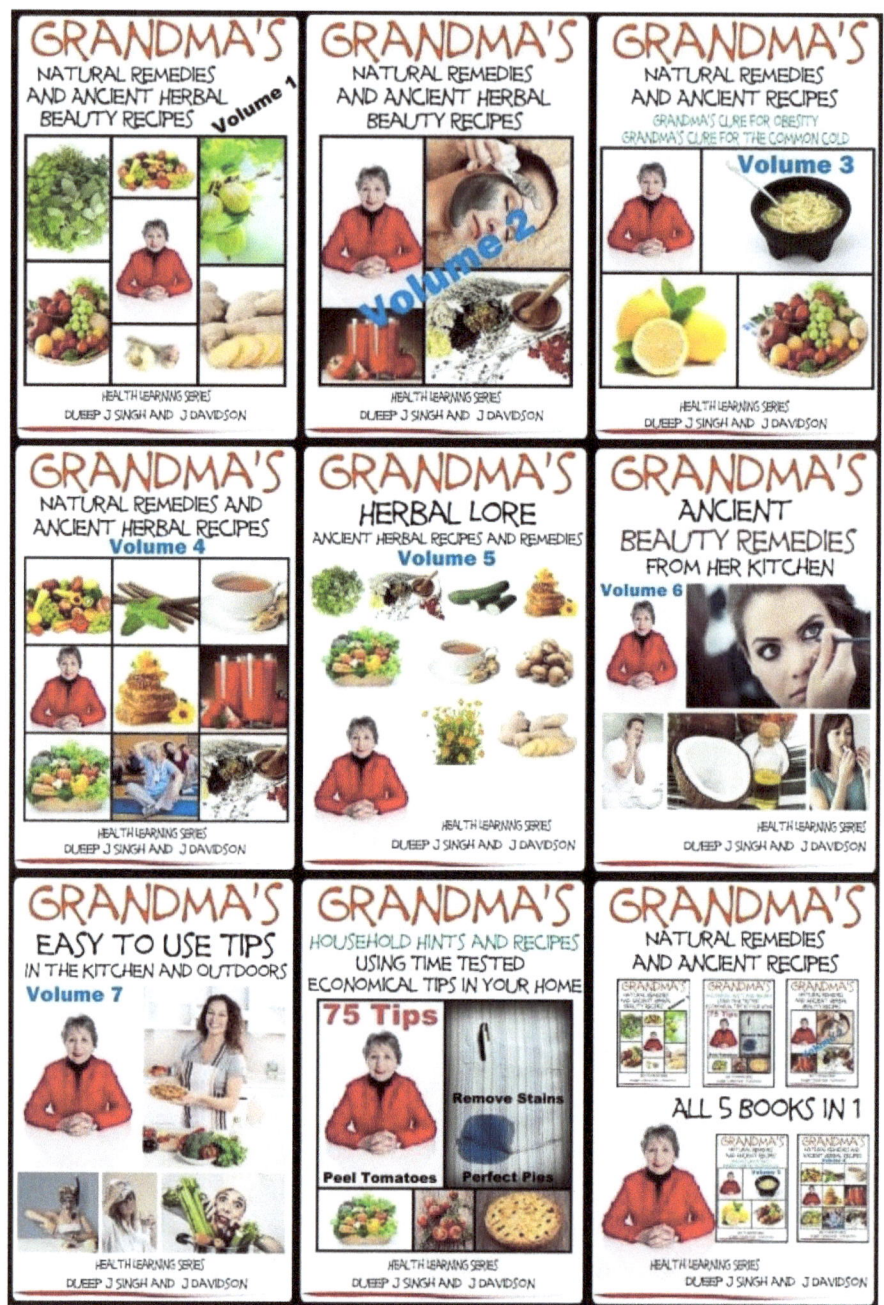

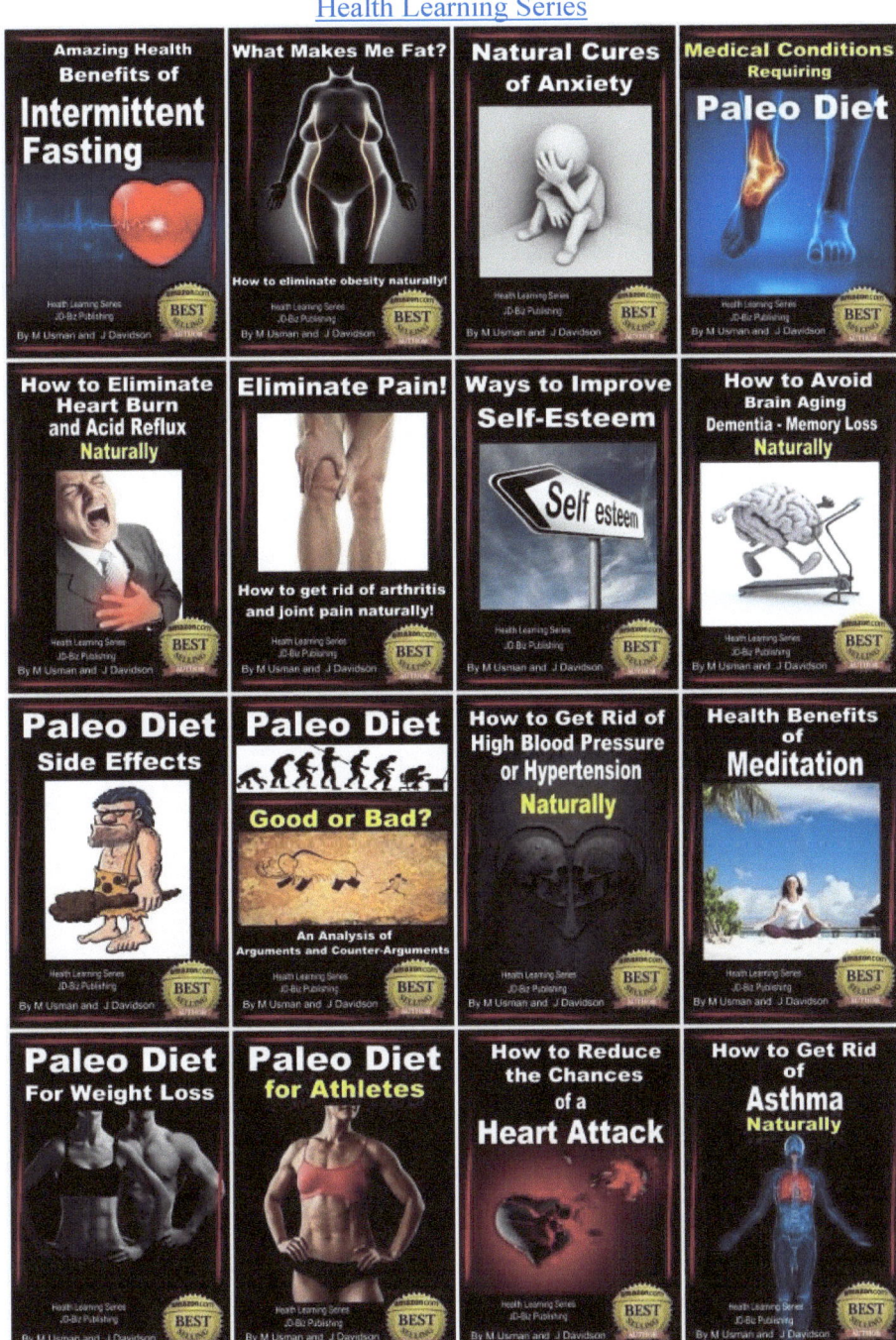

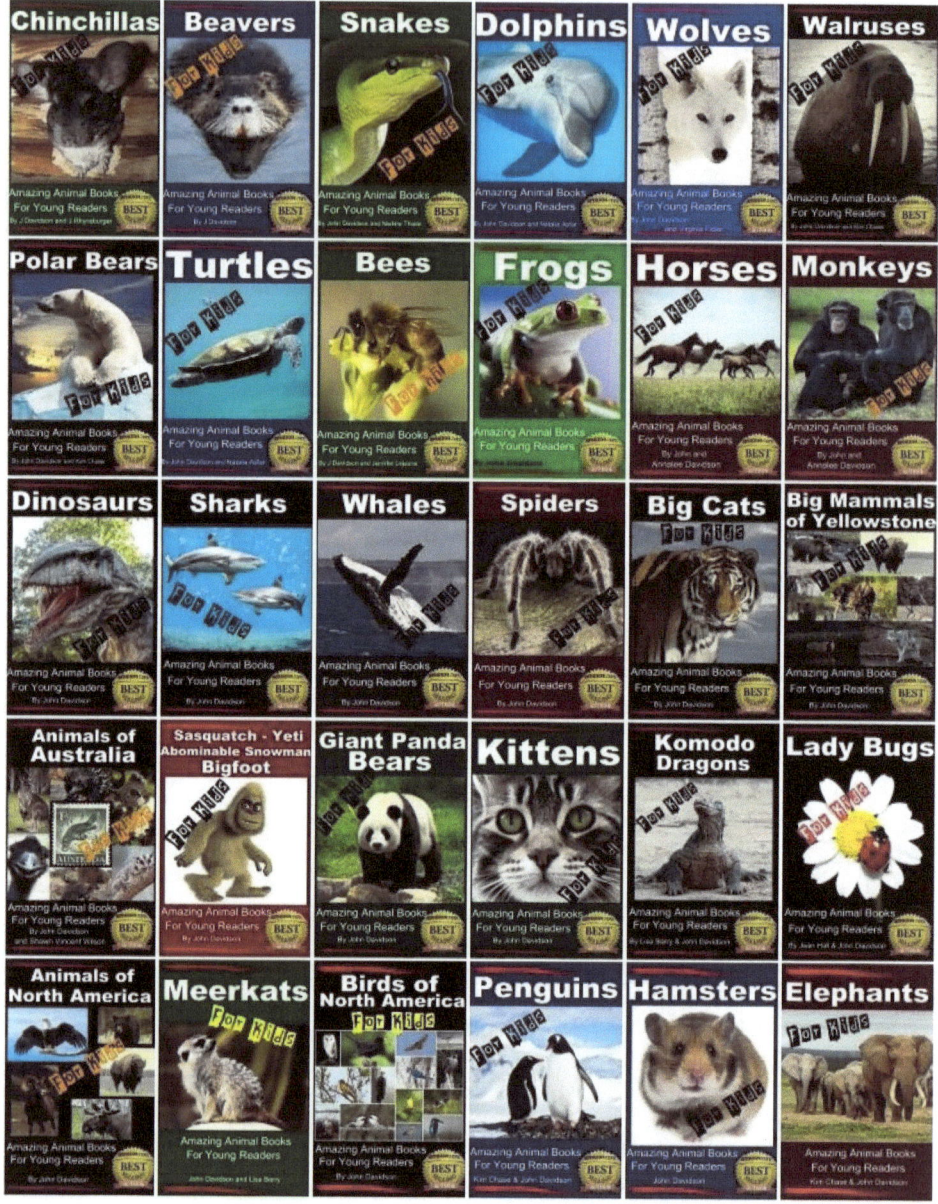

Learn To Draw Series

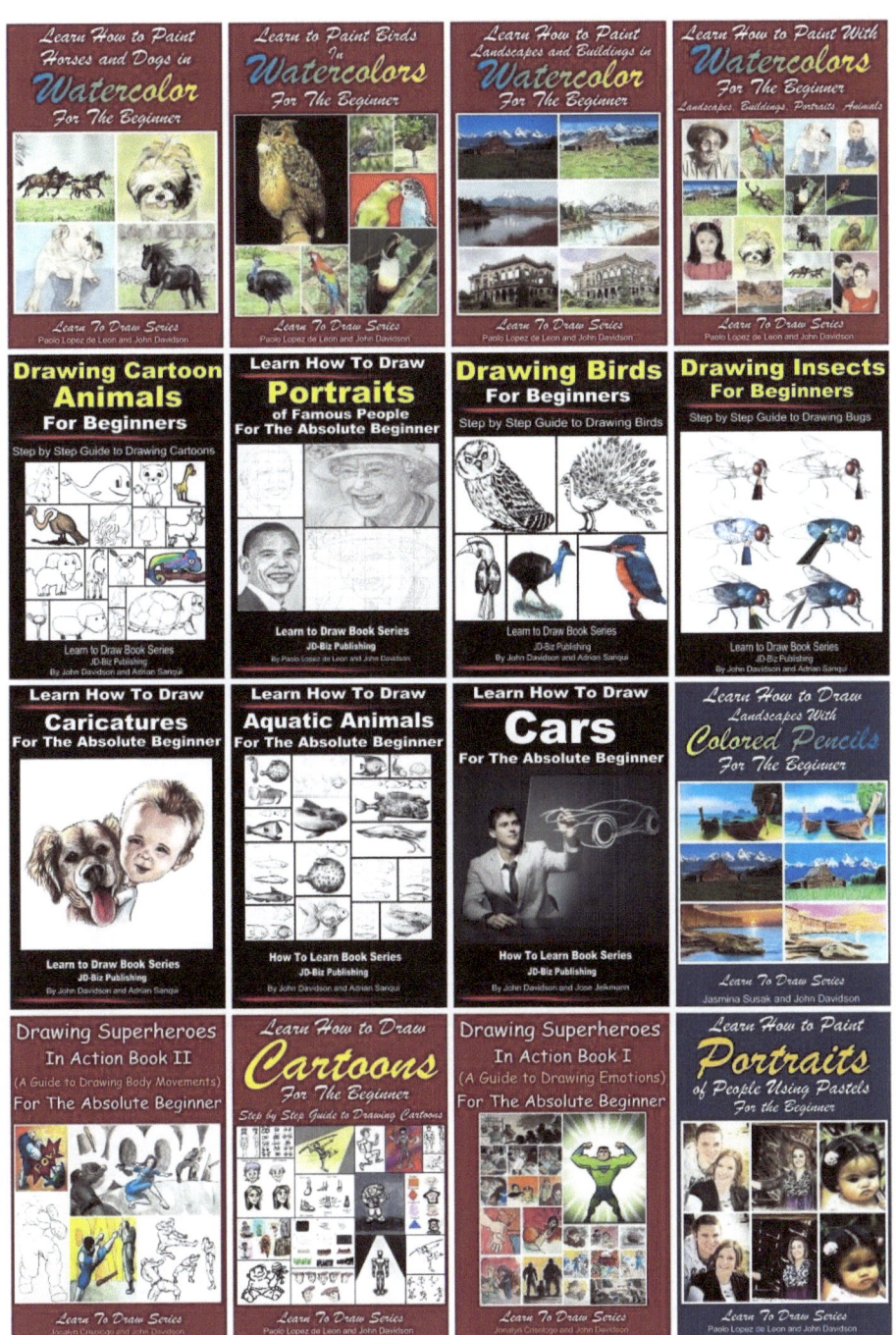

How to Build and Plan Books

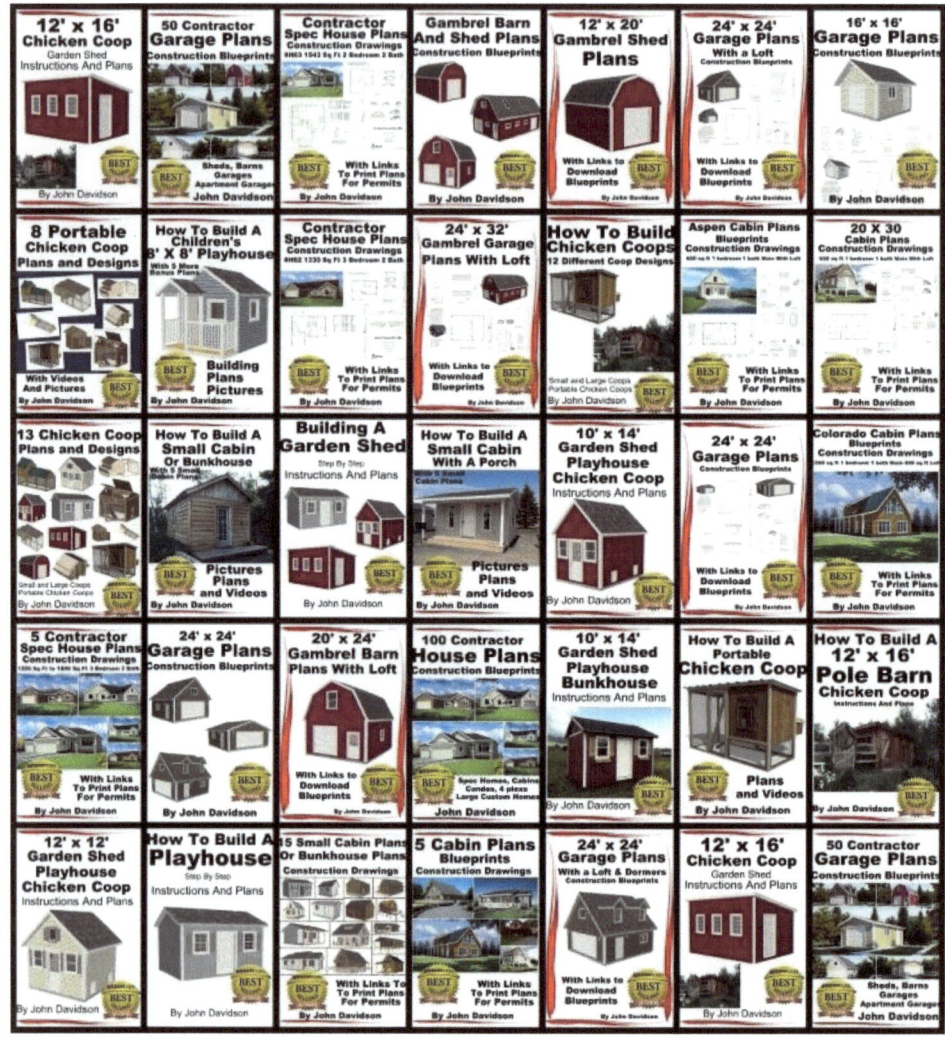

Entrepreneur Book Series

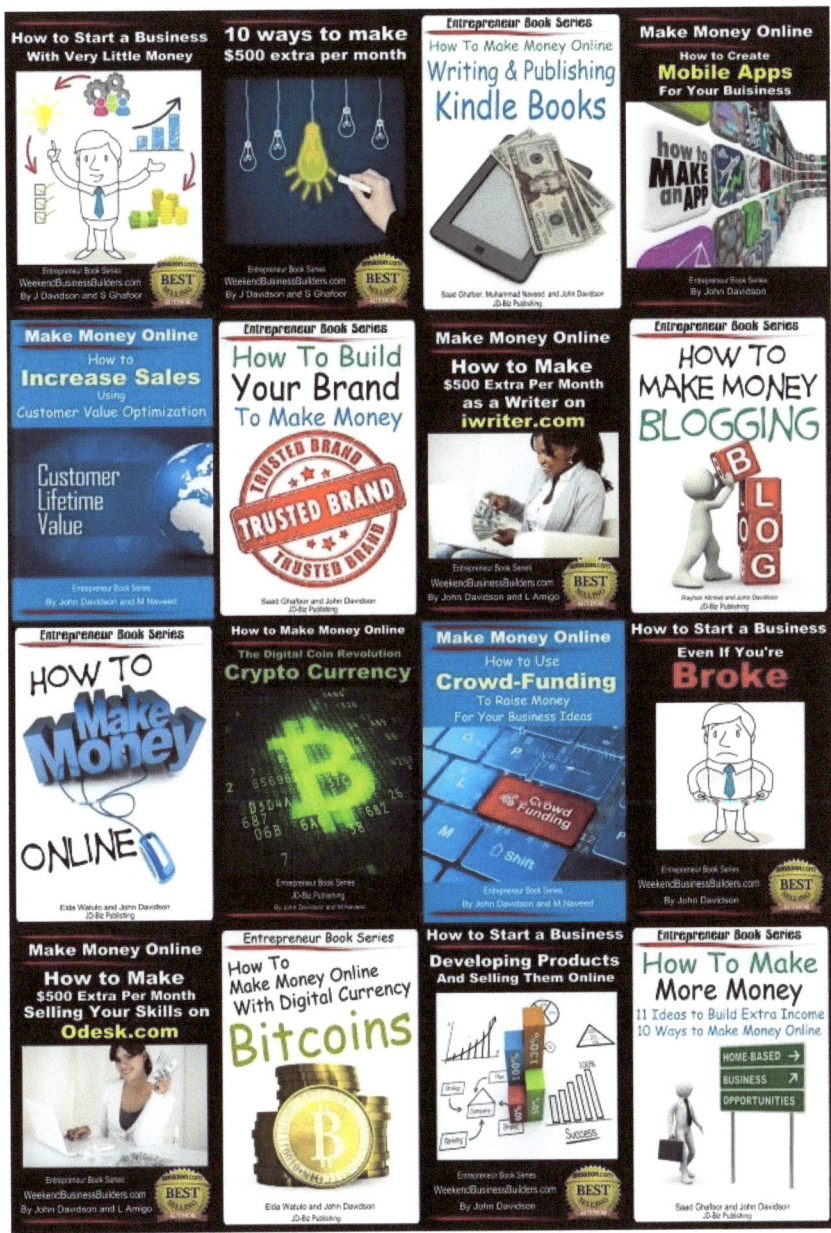

Our books are available at

1. Amazon.com

2. Barnes and Noble

3. Itunes

4. Kobo

5. Smashwords

6. Google Play Books

Download Free Books!

http://MendonCottageBooks.com

Publisher

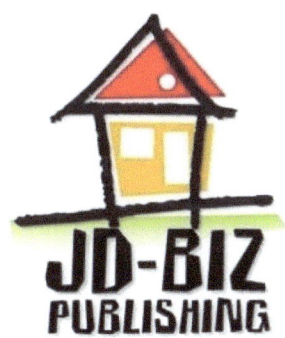

JD-Biz Corp

P O Box 374

Mendon, Utah 84325

http://www.jd-biz.com/

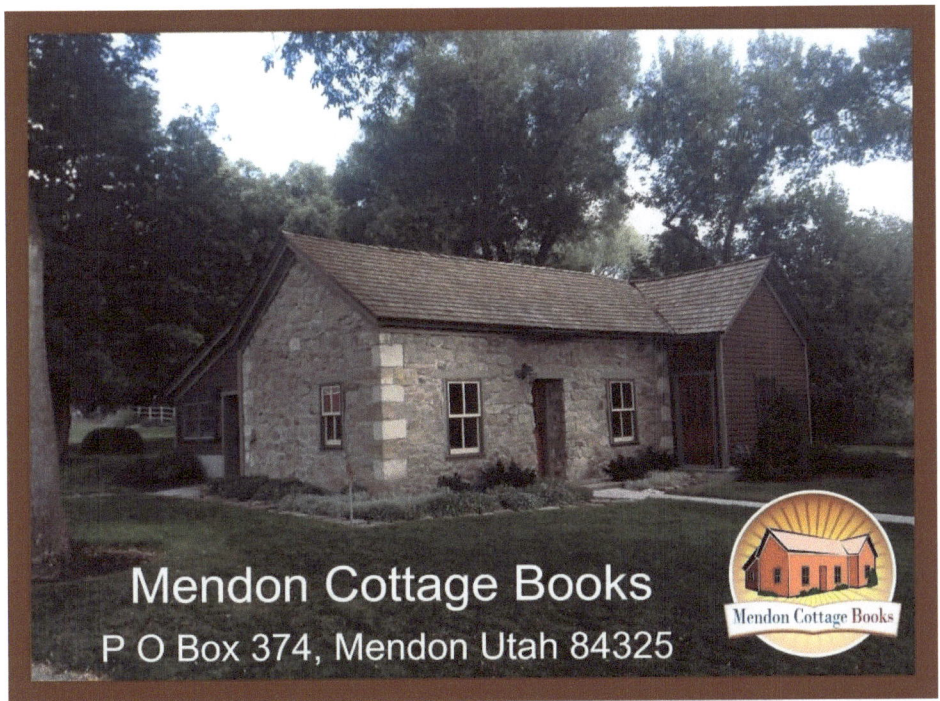